About the author:

I have probably been an addict my entire life, long before I ever picked up a drink or drug. There were times that I wished it was genetic simply to help me understand why I was the way I am. However, neither of my parents were addicts and despite them liking to enjoy a drink or a little weed from time to time.

I have learned over the years that addiction is far more than abuse/lack of control with substances, it relates to poor thinking. I used to joke that I was addicted to everything from Sashimi to my truck. Now the big difference being "addicted" to food and addicted to opiates. Oxy back when they were real, heroin or even the methadone that I tried to use to help me quit. Crack to help me get out of bed in the morning or the overwhelming desire to go gambling that seemed to come with the smoking of rock. Now I am nearly 12 years out from my Opiate addiction, but I have been battling other demons. My wife and I had started experimenting with Oxy together. At the time we were living in the city, and it was hard to go out to any bars, social outings, etc. without running into oxy everywhere. We both realized that we were addicted the same Monday when we both headed to work and realized that we were both dope sick. My wife just walked away from it at that point dealing with the flu like symptoms the following week. Personally, I thought there was an easier way, which is why I came up with Methadone. This was a huge mistake that not only contributed to my 3-year addiction and contributed to having severe arthritis in my knees at only 30-years old.

The most recent one drug addiction problem kicked off as a response to an Upper Respiratory Infection that had been an issue for months. I had gone through numerous rounds of steroids, but the infection would not go away. One summer day, while I was still battling a chest infection, I was cleaning out our garage. Like a scene out of a cartoon, this giant nitrous bottle the size of a 2-litre soda came rolling out at me. I justified trying it out because I need any amount of temporary relief from my chest infection. At the time I had no idea where it had come from but that didn't stop me from picking it up, testing out if the can was full before putting it in my own mouth and being transported to a land of animation. I was completely caught off guard. I had done nitrous when I was a kid at concerts, but this experience was unlike anything I had felt ever before. I later learned that Nitrous works off your opioid receptors so since I had been an opioid addict years before, it successfully knocked me on my ass. That first week I lost 3 days of work before waking back up to the point that I was able to go and speak to my wife to tell her that I had another drug problem and needed to get away for a few days to dry out. I left the US and headed to a British territory where I knew

Nitrous had been banned for sale. I ended up relapsing 9-times the following year before I finally found myself in a residential rehab program in the Pocono mountains. The most frustrating part of this addiction was that I wouldn't even remember my relapses or any portion of drug use apart from waking up in my truck often days later with tanks everywhere. Slowly over the year, Xanax was added to the mix. In the peak of my use, I was going through 10-15 thousand grams of nitrous per day and upwards of 8-9 one milligram Xanax pills.

I am currently clean, I won't even have a drink, I plan on continuing this for many years to come.

Thoughts:

- Need to define the problem before one can work on a solution.

Albert Einstein reportedly said that if he had an hour to solve a problem, he'd spend 55 minutes thinking about the problem and five minutes thinking about solutions. But Einstein wasn't trying to run a company in the midst of a pandemic, when most of us are [working longer hours](#) and making new decisions each day on issues from childcare to employee safety. Between our [cognitive biases](#) and our [finite capacity](#) for decision making, when our mental gas tank runs low on fuel, we tend to conserve energy by either avoiding decisions or rushing to solutions before we have a chance to fully understand the problem we're grappling with.

It's understandable that we leap to solutions. Crossing items of one's to-do list and fixing problems provides a dopamine surge that is comforting, especially when the world around us feels more volatile and threatening. Nevertheless, an ineffective Band-Aid solution can make things worse, and can be just as damaging in the long run as the problem it's trying to solve. In my work as a leadership consultant, I've devised a simple, four-step process that can help you get past the urge to rush to solutions.

1. Go and See

It's easy to jump to lousy solutions when you don't have a strong grasp of the facts — and you can't get that if you don't leave your desk, your office, or your conference room. Gathering facts comes from close observation.

Spreadsheets and reports, which we often rely on are just data, two-dimensional representations of reality. Data tells you how often a machine breaks down on an assembly line. Facts — meaning direct observations — show you that the machine is dirty, covered in oil, and hasn't been cleaned or maintained in a long time.

Data tells you that workers are not on time for their Zoom meetings. Facts — garnered from interviews with your employees — reveal that 9:00am meetings are tough because parents are getting their kids settled for online school; 12:30pm meetings are challenging because they're making lunch for their kids; and that the headlong rush to videoconferencing has all but eliminated the necessary downtime between meetings, and people just need some time for rest.

Data without facts gives you a two-dimensional, black-and-white view of the world. Facts without data give you color and texture, but not the detailed insight you'll need to solve the thorniest problems. Therefore, to arrive at useful conclusions, take both into consideration.

2. Frame Your Problem Properly

Problem statements are deceptively difficult to get right for several reasons. For one, it's easy to mistake the symptoms for the underlying problem. For example, you might assume that to help a child in Flint, Michigan who has behavioral issues in school and struggles with reading comprehension, you need to focus on those problems. But those are only symptoms. The real problem is in the municipal water system.

A well-framed problem statement opens up avenues of discussion and options. A bad problem statement closes down alternatives and quickly sends you into a cul-de-sac of facile thinking.

Consider these two problem statements:

1. Our hospital needs more ventilators.

2. Our hospital needs more ventilator availability.

Notice that the first statement isn't really a problem at all. It's a solution. The only possible response to needing more ventilators is … to buy more ventilators. What's the solution to the second problem statement? It's unclear — which is a good thing, because it pushes us to think more deeply. Avoiding the implicit judgment (we need more machines) raises questions that help us develop better solutions: How many machines are currently being repaired? Are we doing enough preventative maintenance to keep all of them operable? Do we know where all of the ventilators are, or do nurses keep some of them in "hidden stashes" ([a real problem at most hospitals](#)). What's the turnaround time to move a ventilator from one patient to the next? Do other local hospitals have excess capacity, and is it possible to share with them?

If you see that your problem statement has only one solution, rethink it. Begin with observable facts, not opinions, judgments, or interpretations.

3. Think Backwards

When facing a problem, instead of leaping forward toward a solution, go backwards to map out how you got here in the first place.

This fishbone diagram, also known as the Ishikawa diagram, provides a model for identifying potential factors causing your problem:

Use a Fishbone Diagram to Get to Root Causes

Start with the problem and work backward.

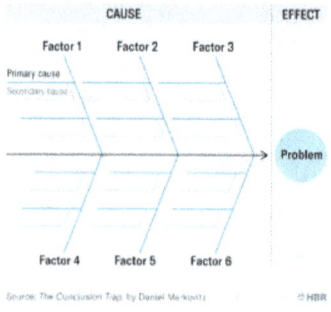

Source: The Conclusion Trap, by Daniel Markovitz   ©HBR

The classic fishbone diagram has six categories of factors, but this isn't a rule; you might have four categories or seven, and your categories might be different. Think of them as prompts to help you organize your thoughts. A law firm, for example, probably won't need the equipment category, while a software company might want to include a branch for programming language.

An Example of a Fishbone Diagram

What are the causes of low morale?

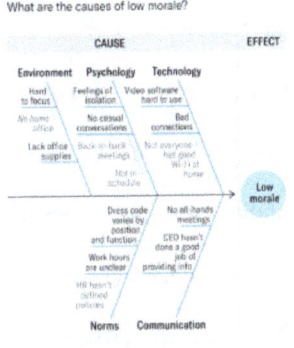

Source: The Conclusion Trap, by Daniel Markovitz

If your firm is struggling with lower morale and employee engagement during the pandemic, you might group contributing factors into the following categories: Work Environment, Technology, Psychology, Communication, and Norms. These prompts will lead you to examine how challenging it is for people to work from home; how well your collaboration software (and people's computer equipment) supports group work; how effectively the company creates opportunities for people to connect with coworkers; how well leadership's messages reach employees; and what cultural norms and expectations are applicable to a work from home reality.

4. Ask Why

Asking "why" repeatedly before you settle on an answer is a powerful way to avoid jumping to conclusions or implementing weak solutions. Whether you ask five times, or three, or as many as 11, eventually you'll get to the root cause, as each question pushes you to a deeper understanding of the real problem. Finding the root cause ensures that you have a durable solution, not a Band-Aid that treats the symptoms. For example, asking, "Why aren't our employees wearing the mandated PPE all the time?" might reveal that you don't have enough PPE in stock, because of a holdup in purchasing. The obvious — and ineffective — solution would be to send a stern memo to the purchasing department instructing them to expedite shipments. But a deeper inquiry with further "whys" would reveal that suppliers weren't delivering on time because the accounting team was stretching out payments in order to conserve cash. . . at the direction of the CEO.

As H.L. Mencken said, "For every complex problem, there is a solution that is clear, simple, and wrong." These four steps don't actually guarantee a solution. But they will provide you with a more clearly defined problem. And although that's less immediately gratifying, it's a necessary step to finding something that really works.

- Need to be able to laugh at yourself. Chances are you have made a series of poor choices that resulted in your current position. Laugh at yourself instead of being awkward and over sensitive.
- Need to focus on yourself (health.)
- You can start your day over at any time.
- LIVE a new life.
- (If you are) dwelling on a problem, you need to share it out loud to hear how dumb it may be.
- Some of the people in rehab are surprisingly brilliant. This one kid (20 years old) was an underwater welder and therefore had to be underwater for 6 to 10 hours a day. This guy figured out a way that he could smoke meth underwater. Now that is engineering. If even a quarter of the effort to get high was used to stay sober/clean, you would live a very successful life.
- You can take away the drug/drink, but you cannot take away the behavior.
- Chart of the brain:

THE DOPAMINERGIC PATHWAYS OF THE BRAIN

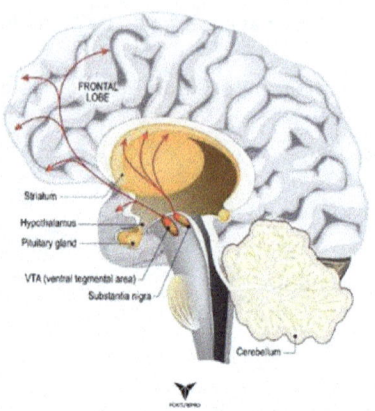

- EMDR and Brain spotting are two therapies used to treat psychological concerns, primarily trauma therapy and PTSD12.The main differences between EMDR and Brain spotting are:

EMDR involves rapid eye movement from right to left or up and down, while Brain spotting usually uses a single eye position.

In EMDR, the eye movements are bilateral and continuous, moving back and forth as a traumatic memory is recalled. In Brain spotting, the therapist will concentrate on the specific locations that the patient's eye moves to and focuses on by itself.

- Edwin Throckmorton Thacher (29 April 1896 – 21 March 1966) (commonly known as Ebby Thacher or Ebby T.) was an old drinking friend and later the sponsor of Alcoholics Anonymous co-founder Bill Wilson. He is credited with introducing Wilson to the initial principles that AA would soon develop, such as "one alcoholic talking to another," and the Jungian thesis which was passed along to Rowland Hazard and, in turn, to Thacher that alcoholics could recover by a "genuine conversion".
- Helping other people stay sober helps me stay sober.
- Alcohol/Drugs are the solution to false needs.
- How can I better understand another person?
- Neurosyphilis occurs when syphilis spreads to the central nervous system. It can happen at any stage of the infection, causing a host of psychiatric and physical symptoms ranging from headaches, personality changes, and loss of coordination to delirium, visual changes, and loss of bladder control…Note: add STDs in addiction info to this section.
- The diagnosis of neurosyphilis is based largely on a lumbar puncture ("spinal tap") and an evaluation of cerebrospinal fluid (CSF). Neurosyphilis can be treated in a hospital with multiple daily doses of penicillin G administered for up to 14 days.

- Methadone is often used to help treat opioid dependence, but it can also cause withdrawal symptoms.

Replacing a drug your body has become dependent on with a prescription medication is a part of recovery known as medication-assisted treatment.

By using one drug to replace another, you can often treat withdrawal symptoms, dependency cravings, and habit-forming effects in the brain.

Methadone is a common choice for medication-assisted treatment. Even though it can be habit-forming, when used correctly, it can help you overcome more intense drug dependencies.

What is methadone and how does it work?

Methadone is an opioid medication that's used to treat severe pain. It's also commonly used to treat dependence to other opioids, like oxycodone and heroin.

Your doctor may prescribe methadone if you need relief from chronic (long-term) pain, or if no other pain medications have made a difference.

Like all opioids, methadone's origins can be traced back to opium, a product of the poppy plant.

Used for thousands of years as a form of pain relief, opium eventually gave rise to commercial medications, like morphine and fentanyl.

All opioids work by binding to certain nerve receptors in the brain, spinal cord, and other areas of the body. These receptors, called opioid receptors, are linked to the body's pain and stress response.

When you take an opioid medication like methadone, the drug binds to those nerve receptors and blocks pain signals.

Many opioid medications also create a feeling of calm and sometimes euphoria, which is part of the reason they can lead to dependence.

While methadone can cause dependence, its long-acting effects are what also help prevent physical withdrawal.

If your body has become dependent on another opioid medication, your healthcare team may prescribe methadone to help you break that cycle of dependency.

Effects of Nitrous Oxide Addiction

1. Physical Health Impacts:
    - Neurological Damage: Chronic use can lead to significant neurological impairments, including nerve damage and numbness, due to the depletion of vitamin B12. This can result in severe, sometimes irreversible conditions like myeloneuropathy, characterized by weakness and difficulty walking 【15】【16】【17】.
    - Respiratory Issues: Using nitrous oxide without oxygen can cause hypoxia, where the body doesn't get enough oxygen. This can lead to

serious complications, including unconsciousness and potentially fatal brain damage 【16】【18】.

- Other Physical Effects: Users often experience weight loss, slurred speech, and difficulty with motor coordination 【16】.

2. Mental Health Consequences:
    - Psychological Effects: Nitrous oxide abuse can lead to paranoia, hallucinations, memory loss, and even psychosis. These effects are particularly concerning due to the gas's ability to alter reality perception, which can be exacerbated by withdrawal 【15】【17】.
    - Addiction and Dependence: The quick onset and short duration of nitrous oxide's euphoric effects often lead to repeated use, increasing the risk of dependence. Over time, higher doses are required to achieve the same effect, which can lead to a dangerous cycle of addiction 【17】【18】.

Personal Experiences and Recovery Strategies

Including your personal experiences with the severe weight loss, paranoia, and hallucinations will provide a powerful narrative that highlights the real dangers of nitrous oxide abuse. It's also essential to discuss the role of strong anti-psychotic medications in your recovery, offering readers insight into potential treatments and the seriousness of the condition.

Alternative Recovery Programs: Dharma and SMART Recovery

- Dharma Recovery: This program integrates Buddhist teachings and practices, focusing on mindfulness, meditation, and the Four Noble Truths to help individuals manage cravings and understand the nature of addiction.
- SMART Recovery: Offers a secular, science-based approach to recovery, emphasizing self-empowerment and self-reliance. It provides tools and techniques for self-directed change, helping individuals build and maintain motivation, manage emotions, and develop healthier lifestyles.

These alternative approaches may appeal to those seeking different methods than traditional 12-step programs, providing diverse strategies for achieving and maintaining sobriety.

Short Stories:

The director of this rehab was telling a story about his struggle with recovery. There was a point where his sponsor called him a Firetruck and he dismissed it. The sponsor then called him a POS where he immediately became defensive. The reason is because he believes that he is a piece of shit.

Daily Matras/Prayers:

- More you, less me.
- Need to keep my side of the street clean.

Random Facts:

- Giraffes are 30x more likely to be struck by lightning than humans.
- Obesity is a result of malnutrition. Note: Expand on.
- Human teeth are the only body part that cannot heal itself.
- Flamingos aren't born pink.
- Elephants cannot jump.
- Residential treatment (rehab) used to be 1-year long.
- Addicts hate two things, 1) Change, 2) Things how they are.
- Hawaiian pizza was invented in Canada.

Quotes:

- "Truth is always exciting…life is dull without it." – Paul S Buck
- "The soul is healed by being with children." – Dostoyevsky
- "Two things I beat, the Odds & my Meat." – Bumper Sticker
- "I couldn't wait for success, so I went ahead without it." – John Winters
- "Everyman takes the limits of his own field of vision for the limits of the world." – Arnold Schwarzenegger
- The young man knows the rules, the old man knows how to break them.

Advice:

- Life is just a series of questions/choices. Choice is POWER.
- Get out of your own head, its like being stuck in a bad neighborhood.
- You don't need to be too hard on yourself, chances are you have a mother/spouse for that.
- Substance abuse is not necessarily a substance problem, its thinking problem.
- Be aware of your surroundings.

- It is easy to ask for help, it is much harder to accept and implement said advice.
- Don't be braggadocious.
- Just move your body, it helps with every area of health.
- Evaluate what you are willing to do to life/stay sober. Compare the list to what you did/are still willing to do to get high.
- You can catch a monkey with a wicker basket with a small opening and some food. The monkey will reach in to grab the food but won't be able to remove the arm afterwards. They will refuse to release the food even if it means that are trapped.
- Rule #62 – "Don't take yourself too seriously."

Acronyms:

FINE – Fucked up, Insecure, Neurotic, & Emotional.

FEAR –

- Fucked Everything and Run,
- Fight Everyone and Relapse,
- False Evidence Appearing Real,

- Face Everything and Recover.

PUSH – Pray until something happens.

FAMILY – Forget About Me, I Love You.

Staying Sober: Avoid having to explain your sobriety.

- At restaurants, flipping the empty wine glass upside down on the table lets the staff know that you do not drink and will not require the drink menu.
- "Friend of Bill W" is a statement saying that you are in recovery.
- Many locations that do not have a formal 12-step meeting (Ex. A cruise ship) will allow a "party for Bill W" so that people in recovery have a safe place to meet daily.
- Announcements for the "friends of Bill W," common in airports and other transportation locations, alert members that someone is struggling and needs help.
- "417" is a code for Acceptance. The number comes from the page in the Big Book on acceptance.
- "Wart rats" is a common name for groups of people in recovery and are common at music festivals.
- Yellow balloons and/or flags may also signify sober areas at sports venues, concerts, etc.
- If you are attending a concert, check the Facebook account of the band. It is common for them to have a sober group of fans that are always open to new people joining.

Who I Was? Open Ended Questions:

- Ask yourself-
    - What did I look like when I was actively using?
    - What was I being told about myself when I was using?
    - What did individuals tell me I looked like when I was using?
    - What are the short/long term effects of my using?
    - Who has been affected by my using?

Definition:

Pro re neta – as the need arises

Glutamate - the most abundant excitatory neurotransmitter released by nerve cells in your brain. It plays a major role in learning and memory. For your brain to function properly, glutamate needs to be present in the right concentration in the right places at the right time. Too much glutamate is associated with such diseases as Parkinson's disease, Alzheimer's disease and Huntington's disease.

Anhedonia - the inability to experience joy or pleasure. You may feel numb or less interested in things that you once enjoyed. It's a common symptom of many mental health conditions like depression. Treatment is available to help you regain interest in life's activities, like being around loved ones or listening to music.

Dry Goods – What drugs are referred to in AA.

S.M.A.R.T. – Self Management and Recovery Training. The program is evidence based.

G.O.D. – Good orderly direction.

Positive Action – Any action that leaves you with a good feeling.

Agnostic – Don't believe, don't not believe.

H.A.L.T. – Hungry, Angry, Lonely, Tired.

Psychosis - a combination of symptoms resulting in an impaired relationship with reality. It can be a symptom of serious [mental health disorders](). People who are experiencing psychosis may have either hallucinations or delusions.

[Hallucinations]() are sensory experiences that occur within the absence of an actual stimulus. For example, a person having an auditory hallucination may hear their mother yelling at them when their mother isn't around. Or someone having a visual hallucination may see something, like a person in front of them, who isn't there.

The person experiencing psychosis may also have thoughts that are contrary to actual evidence. These thoughts are known as delusions. Some people with psychosis may also experience loss of motivation and social withdrawal.

These experiences can be frightening. They may also cause people who are experiencing psychosis to hurt themselves or others.

It's important to get medical help right away if you or someone else is experiencing symptoms of psychosis.

Nephrotic syndrome - a kidney disorder that causes your body to pass too much protein in your urine.

Nephrotic syndrome is usually caused by damage to the clusters of small blood vessels in your kidneys that filter waste and excess water from your blood. The condition causes swelling, particularly in your feet and ankles, and increases the risk of other health problems.

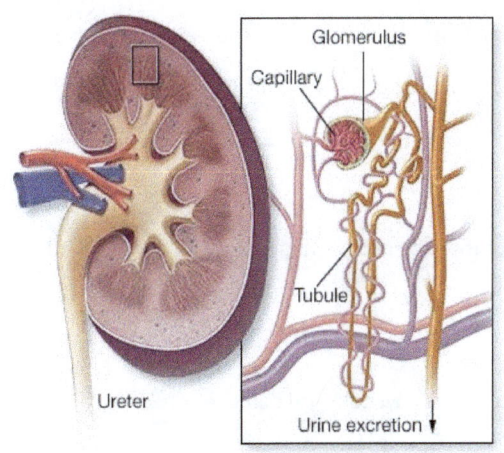

What are Cognitive Distortions?

Cognitive distortions are biased perspectives we take on ourselves and the world around us. They are irrational thoughts and beliefs that we unknowingly reinforce over time.

These patterns and systems of thought are often subtle—it's difficult to recognize them when they are a regular feature of your day-to-day thoughts. That is why they can be so damaging since it's hard to change what you don't recognize as something that needs to change!

Cognitive distortions come in many forms (which we'll cover later in this piece), but they all have some things in common.

All cognitive distortions are:

- Tendencies or patterns of thinking or believing.

- That are false or inaccurate.

- And have the potential to cause psychological damage.

It can be scary to admit that you may fall prey to distorted thinking. You might be thinking, "There's no way I am holding on to any blatantly false beliefs!" While most people don't suffer in their daily lives from these kinds of cognitive distortions, it seems that no one can completely escape these distortions.

If you're human, you have likely fallen for a few of the numerous cognitive distortions at one time or another. The difference between those who occasionally stumble into a cognitive distortion and those who struggle with them on a more long-term basis is the ability to identify and modify or correct these faulty patterns of thinking.

As with many skills and abilities in life, some are far better at this than others—but with practice, you can improve your ability to recognize and respond to these distortions.

These distortions have been shown to relate positively to symptoms of depression, meaning that where cognitive distortions abound, symptoms of depression are likely to occur as well (Burns, Shaw, & Croker, 1987).

In the words of the renowned psychiatrist and researcher David Burns:

"I suspect you will find that a great many of your negative feelings are in fact based on such thinking errors."

Errors in thinking, or cognitive distortions, are particularly effective at provoking or exacerbating symptoms of depression. It is still a bit ambiguous as to whether these distortions cause depression or depression brings out these distortions (after all, correlation does not equal causation!) but they frequently go together.

Johari Window:

- The Johari Window is a framework you and your team can use to develop better self-awareness of your conscious and unconscious biases.

- You can use it to compare what you consider to be your own strengths and weaknesses to others' perceptions of them.

- The Johari Window is split into four quadrants: the Open Area (things you know about yourself), the Blind Area (things you don't know about yourself, but others do), the Hidden Area (things you know about yourself, but keep hidden), and the Unknown Area (things that are unknown to you and to others).

- You can use the Johari Window in your organization to build trust, develop self-awareness, and improve understanding and interpersonal relationships with your colleagues.

A.V.R.T.: The Addictive Voice Recognition Technique is a practice used in Rational Recovery to help individuals recognize and resist the "addictive voice" – the thoughts and urges that justify or encourage substance use. By objectively recognizing these thoughts as AV, individuals can abstain from addictive behaviors.

Wet brain: A disorder of the brain caused by a chronic thiamine (vitamin B1) deficiency. It's also known as Wernicke-Korsakoff syndrome (WKS), named after German neurologist Carl Wernicke and neuropsychiatrist Sergei Korsakoff.

WKS can be divided into two stages or conditions: Wernicke's encephalopathy and Korsakoff's psychosis. Wet brain is most seen in people with alcohol use disorder. In fact, the term 'wet brain' was developed in direct reference to the condition's link with alcohol dependence and misuse.

While anyone can develop the disorder, people who consume alcohol are more likely to develop the condition. According to the National Institute on Alcohol Abuse and Alcoholism, 80% of people with alcohol use disorder have a thiamine deficiency.

Research shows that wet brain is more likely to develop in men than women. This is because men are more likely to be diagnosed with alcohol use disorder, the leading cause of wet brain. With the proper treatment and management, it's possible to reverse the damage the condition has caused to your brain.

Periodic Table of Intoxicates:

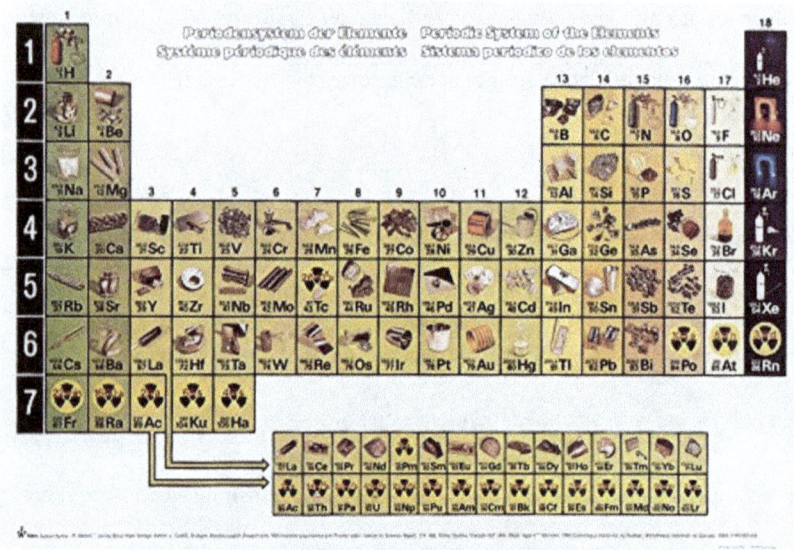

Joke(s):

If you want to make God laugh, tell him your plan.

Thoughts:

AA/NA is the only place where you can publicly announce how you just blew your entire life up and everybody claps for you. It's insane.

What I learned in Residential Treatment (Rehab):

I can only truly make amends to the loved ones that I have hurt over the years by staying sober.

AA was started by Doctor Bob & Bill W in 1935. NA started in 1953. Currently there are over 100 different 12-step programs. Ebby was the first person to share her story.

Get/retain buffers to ensure your sobriety.

Shut the fuck up and listen to what other people have to say.

I am a stubborn asshole.

Be mindful of your audience.

Be aware of what works for you.

We cannot change the past but we can use that shame/guilt as a motivator to stay clean.

Addicts have an allergy to D&A, similar to an allergy to peanuts or cats.

Nothing is impossible, not by miracles, but by hard work and a structured plan.

Live life like a loved one is always standing next to you.

The strong will carry the weak.

Ideal times are dangerous.

M^2 – Opioid receptors.

You do not know another person's traumas.

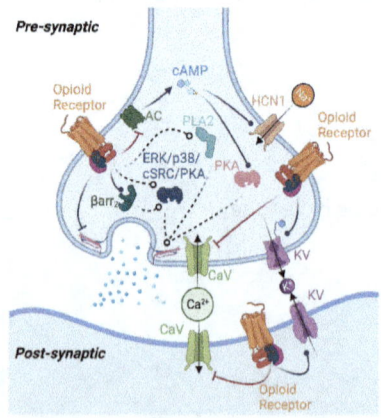

Pointing out other people's problems or defects is a form of Deflecting.

Do not be concerned with People Pleasing.

An apology without a change is meaningless.

Trust is a two-way street.

Progress starts at your pace.

I want to live today/tomorrow.

Do not Assassinate Characters.

Together "we" stay sober, alone "I" get high.

Stop Projecting Thoughts.

Do not Project Problems.

I have a history of completing blowing up my life every few years.

Sobriety will only work if I do it for myself, not for other people.

Be careful about sharing your emotions in the program unless you are ready to welcome hugs (support) by 100+ people.

Note: See "Last Run."

10 Indicative Signs You're Ready to Get Sober

By David Beasley

Publish Date: September 24, 2023

Medically Reviewed by: Charley Allen

Addiction, whether it's alcohol misuse or substance abuse, is a complex disease that impacts both your mental and physical health. It can creep in subtly, often unrecognized, until its consequences are hard to ignore.

By understanding and recognizing the signs indicating readiness to quit drinking or drug use, you take the first step toward a healthier and more fulfilling life.

Sign #1: Acknowledgment of the Problem

Sign 1 Acknowledgment of the Problem Design for Recovery

The first sign you're ready to get sober is admitting to yourself that you have a problem. This step requires introspection and honesty. This admission signifies the pivotal shift from denial to acceptance, and it requires asking some tough questions:

"Has my drug or alcohol use negatively impacted my life?"

"Do I feel a constant need to use substances to feel normal?"

"Am I experiencing withdrawal symptoms if I don't use substances?"

"Has my substance use strained my relationships or caused problems at work or school?"

Your sincere answers to these questions are crucial. They can reveal the degree to which substance use has disrupted your life and well-being. Admitting to yourself that you have an addiction problem can be difficult, but it's a step towards reclaiming control of your life.

Part of admitting you have a problem is understanding what getting sober and staying sober means for you. Sobriety isn't just about abstaining from substances. It involves cultivating a new, healthier lifestyle that enables you to cope with life's ups and downs without resorting to drugs or alcohol.

Acknowledging your problem also means understanding that recovery isn't a quick fix. It's not about stopping cold turkey or promising yourself you'll have just one more drink. Recovery is a journey—a commitment to a new way of living that includes developing strategies to remain sober and avoid relapse. It means making significant changes, such as distancing yourself from toxic relationships and seeking professional support when needed.

Acknowledging your problem with substance use is the first indicator that you're ready to pursue a life of sobriety, reclaim control, and return to a more normal life.

Sign #2: Desperation or Hitting Rock Bottom

Sign 2 Desperation or Hitting Rock Bottom Design for Recovery

One of the signs you are ready to get sober is when you reach a point of desperation or hit what many refer to as "rock bottom." This stage is a deeply personal and painful place where the impact of substance use disorder has taken a severe toll on your life, prompting a desperate need for change.

"Rock bottom" isn't a universal concept—it differs for each individual. It's a point in your life when the negative consequences of your drug or alcohol use are so overwhelming that they compel a critical shift in perspective. Your rock bottom could be a culmination of several elements:

Physical health deterioration: You may suffer from constant fatigue, chronic pain, or serious health conditions caused or exacerbated by drug or alcohol use.

Emotional distress: Feelings of depression, anxiety, or other mental health issues linked to substance use have become unbearable.

Relationship breakdowns: Substance use has driven a wedge between you and your family, friends, or partner.

Career and financial problems: Your work performance or financial stability is negatively impacted by your substance use.

Legal issues: You may have gotten into legal trouble due to activities related to your addiction.

Hitting rock bottom is often the wake-up call that prompts you to seek help and get sober. It signals that you're at a point where you can no longer ignore the consequences of your substance use and that you're ready to make significant changes in your life.

When you've reached this critical point, it's important to seek support and treatment facilities to help you on your path to recovery. Experiencing desperation or hitting rock bottom can be a painful realization but also an opportunity. It's a moment of clarity that can spark your decision to get sober and make the necessary changes to recover from your substance use disorder

Sign #3: Strained Relationships

Sign 3 Strained Relationships Design for Recovery

Substance use disorder often strains relationships with family members, friends, and coworkers. If you find your relationships suffer from alcohol or drug use, this can be a sign you're ready to seek professional help.

Substance use disorder often interferes with personal connections, and the desire to mend these strained relationships can be a strong motivating factor in the decision to get sober. The effects of substance use on relationships can manifest in several ways:

Dishonesty: You might find yourself lying about your substance use, which can erode trust in relationships.

Neglect: Substance use can lead to neglecting responsibilities or important events in the lives of those you care about.

Conflict: Frequent arguments or disagreements about your drug or alcohol use can increase tension in your relationships.

Isolation: You might distance yourself from loved ones or prefer to spend time with others who use substances.

Numerous people who have overcome addiction share how their desire to mend or build healthy relationships prompted them to get sober.

Sign #4: Health Concerns

Sign 4 Health Concerns Design for Recovery

Substance use disorders can significantly impact your physical health. The evidence is clear, ranging from severe health conditions like liver disease caused by heavy alcohol use to sleep problems induced by certain substances. Recognizing these health concerns often acts as a potent motivator to stop drinking or using drugs. Many individuals who successfully embarked on their sobriety journey recall a serious health scare as their turning point.

The detrimental health effects of substance use can present in various ways, such as:

Liver disease: Heavy alcohol use can lead to conditions like cirrhosis and alcoholic hepatitis.

Cardiovascular issues: Both drug and alcohol use can increase the risk of heart disease and stroke.

Respiratory problems: Certain drugs, especially when smoked, can cause respiratory issues, including lung disease and breathing problems.

Mental health disorders: Substance use often co-occurs with conditions like depression, anxiety, and other mental health disorders.

Sleep disturbances: Many substances can interfere with normal sleep patterns, leading to insomnia or other sleep disorders.

If you're experiencing any of these health issues, seeking help is crucial.

Sign #5: Financial Difficulties

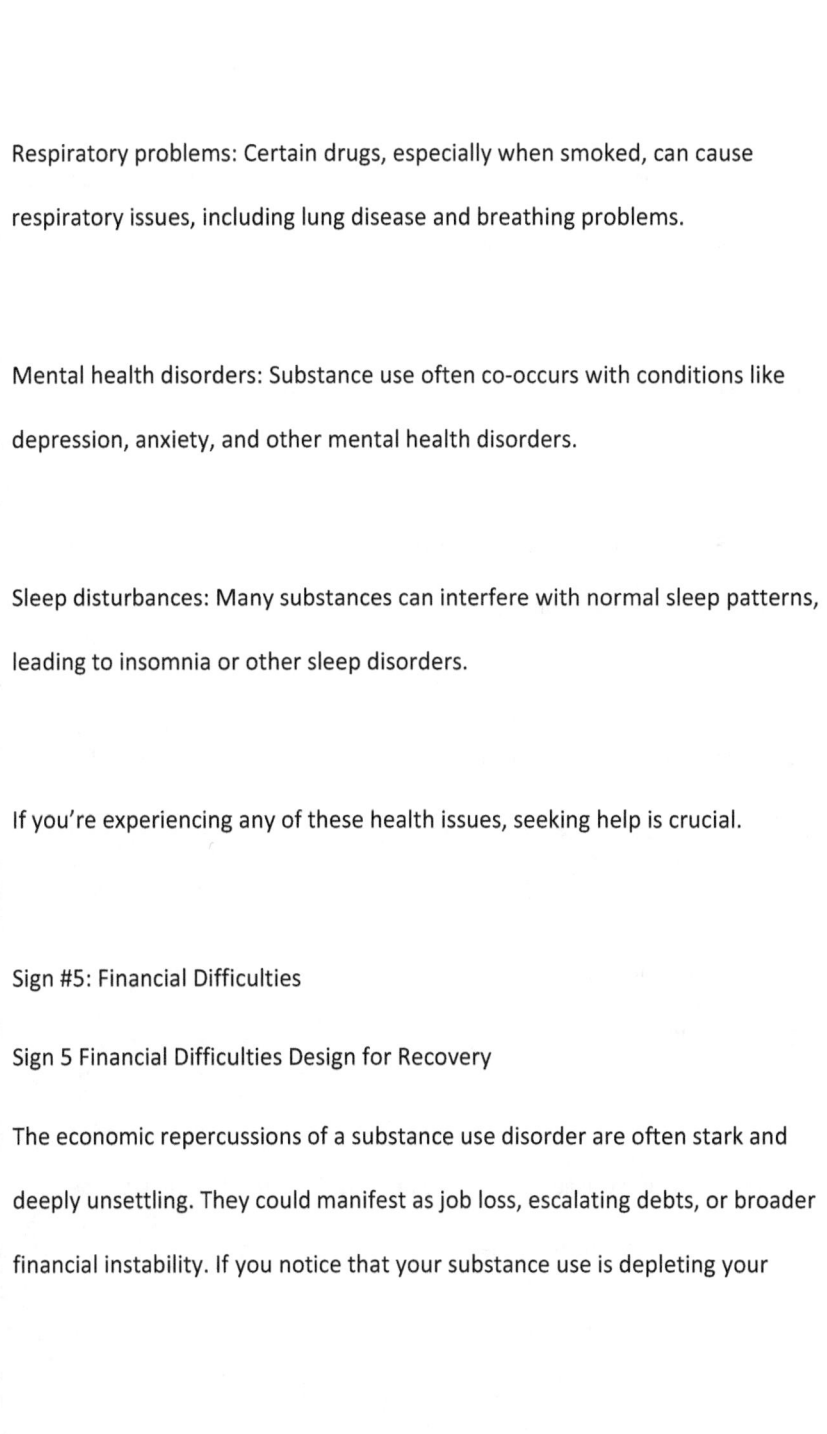

Sign 5 Financial Difficulties Design for Recovery

The economic repercussions of a substance use disorder are often stark and deeply unsettling. They could manifest as job loss, escalating debts, or broader financial instability. If you notice that your substance use is depleting your financial resources or impeding your ability to fulfill your financial obligations, this is a compelling sign that you're ready to seek sobriety.

Substance use could lead to financial hardship in several ways:

Job Loss: Substance use could result in impaired work performance, missed days, or ultimately job termination.

High Costs: Purchasing drugs or alcohol frequently can lead to considerable financial drain.

Legal Fees: Substance use could lead to legal issues, which often result in hefty legal fees or fines.

Neglecting Financial Obligations: Money that should be used for rent, utilities, or other bills may be redirected towards sustaining the addiction.

Legal issues related to drug or alcohol use often serve as critical wake-up calls, prompting individuals to consider sobriety. Legal problems such as Driving Under the Influence (DUI) charges, drug possession offenses, or incidents related to substance-impaired behaviors can drastically affect an individual's life, potentially motivating them to get sober. Many people now leading sober lives cite legal consequences as a primary catalyst for their decision to change.

Legal issues stemming from substance use can vary, including:

Driving Under the Influence (DUI) or Driving While Intoxicated (DWI) charges.

Drug possession or dealing charges.

Legal problems related to behavior under the influence, such as disorderly conduct or physical altercations.

Legal repercussions impacting family life, like child custody disputes.

Legal troubles can be daunting, but they can also act as a forceful motivator for positive change. With the right support network, treatment resources, and personal commitment, these challenges can be the turning point to a sober life. The focus should be on the immediate need to deal with legal issues and the broader objective of sustained sobriety and a healthier lifestyle.

Sign #8: Failed Attempts to Quit

Sign 8 Failed Attempts to Quit Design for Recovery

Failed attempts to quit substance use can be emotionally taxing but can also signify readiness to pursue sobriety. Experiencing a relapse is not unusual; in fact, it's a common component of the recovery journey. According to the National Institute on Drug Abuse, relapse rates for addiction mimic those of other chronic illnesses, such as hypertension and asthma. The crucial point is not to view a relapse as a failure but rather as an indicator that your treatment plan may need fine-tuning.

Understanding the common causes of relapse can be helpful:

Exposure to triggers: Environmental or emotional cues that can cause intense cravings, leading to substance use.

Lack of support: The absence of a supportive network of family, friends, and sober companions can hinder the recovery process.

Insufficient coping mechanisms: Lack of effective coping skills to handle stress and negative emotions can often lead to a relapse.

Inadequate treatment plan: A treatment plan that doesn't fully address an individual's unique needs can result in unsuccessful attempts to quit.

The important message to take from relapses is that they are not a sign of failure but rather a part of the journey to sobriety. They can provide valuable lessons about what works and what doesn't in your personal fight against addiction.

Sign #9: Lack of Interest in Activities Once Enjoyed

Sign 9 Lack of Interest in Activities Once Enjoyed Design for Recovery

Loss of interest in activities that once brought pleasure can be a potent sign that it's time to quit substance use. This shift, often referred to as anhedonia in clinical terms, is frequently seen in people struggling with substance use disorder. It might involve the diminishing joy from hobbies, social events, or even personal relationships that used to be meaningful. If you find yourself longing for the passion you once had for these activities or experiences, it could indicate that you're ready to embark on the journey to sobriety.

Anhedonia occurs due to the impact of chronic substance use on the brain's reward system. The constant influx of substances can overstimulate this system, causing it to become less responsive to natural rewards. Hence, activities that once brought joy no longer have the same effect. However, knowing that this condition is reversible with proper treatment and sustained sobriety is important.

Sign 10: Acceptance of the Need for Help

One of the most significant milestones on the road to sobriety is the acceptance that you can't conquer addiction alone and acknowledging the need for help. This realization is powerful, as it forms the basis for seeking external support in your journey to recovery. It could involve reaching out to a healthcare provider, seeking mental health resources, joining mutual support groups, or enrolling in a formal addiction treatment program.

The Substance Abuse and Mental Health Services Administration (SAMHSA) underscores the indispensable role of support systems in recovery from substance use disorders. Accepting help does not signify weakness; rather, it reflects your strength in recognizing that addiction is a complex issue that requires a multi-faceted approach.

Random Facts:

- The average cloud weighs a 100 million tons.
- Definition of Love is putting the wants and needs before your own.
- Anadreis fault line moves at the same speed that the average person's nails grow.

15 Signs That You Are A Sober Person

When you first enter the wide, wonderful and oftentimes unpredictable world of recovery, there is a definite sense of struggle. Leaving behind the old and destructive ways of addiction and adapting newer and healthier ways of thinking, feeling and acting takes a lot of active practice as well as continual trial and error.

When you take your first baby steps in sobriety, you can feel like you have two left feet and it can feel like you are stumbling around more than actually moving forwards. After awhile the recovery mindset starts to become second nature, and as time progresses we may notice during those random quiet times in our daily routines there are things that you do or say in your recovery that you didn't do when you were active in our substance abuse.

Listed below are 15 signs that you are a sober person.

You Handle Day-to-Day Situations Differently

Let's get down to the nitty gritty, life isn't perfect. In your never-ending recovery journey, you will encounter obstacles and challenges in your everyday life that test the limits of your patience. One of the signs that you a sober person is that you are able to slow down and take what is given to you at face value. As a result, you take what you need and leave the rest.

You Learn to Learn

Let's also face it... life is short–too short. While recovery is something you take seriously, taking yourself seriously 24-7 can actually undermine your recovery in the long run. You will make mistakes and fall short at times. As a sober person, you can take the time to look back at what you accomplished thus far in recovery and the obstacles you've overcome, and realize that with each obstacle that is overcome you grow stronger and more confident that you can overcome the next obstacle that crosses your path.

Focusing on the Positive

Those who assume the role of Negative Nancy are classic examples of folks who display a victim mentality where they assume no responsibility for their standing in life. Guess what? YOU DO! Another one of the signs that you are a sober person is that you get the fact that life happens and while sucky things occur, there are also a lot of upsides of living a sober life.

You Got People

One of the most important signs that you are a sober person is that you have a network of friends, family and peers in recovery you have your back and will extend a hand, shoulder to lean on or an ear to bend when the going gets rough in your recovery. As a sober person sometimes you have to step back and realize the wonderful resources you have at your disposal. Many people, many stories, much wisdom and you drink tons of coffee (more on that later).

You Can Check Yourself

As a sober person the virtue of patience can be one of the most challenging things to cultivate. Sobriety at times can render you like a walking nerve—everything and anything can irritate or aggravate you. However, you have learned an important lesson in your recovery journey and that lesson is simple: let go. You know that you have embrace your life as a person in recovery when you can fully understand the present moment and ultimately realize that how you handle the situation right now will determine how your future can play out.

Coffee!

In sobriety, it seems as though coffee is currency. The smell permeates the meeting room and is the beverage of choice in social gathering where sober folks are present. Even if you don't fancy yourself a coffee drinker you may find yourself drinking quite a bit. (writer's note…I like mine strong with four sugar cubes.)

You Experience Happiness

Yeah, life can be difficult at times and provide a real kick in the pants but comparing it to where you came from all things are relative. Sober folks are generally a happy lot because they are living and breathing and living life on life's terms day by day. Knowing that you hold the key to make things happen in your life is another sign that you are a sober person. Now…get things done!

You Have Principles

Sober people have cultivated some form of spiritual undercurrent that guides their lives. It's doesn't have to be God proper, but those who are sober realize there is a power greater than themselves. Because of that, those who are sober realize they are just a spoke in the wheel. You can try, but your arms are too short to box with God (I have tried, I know...)

You Wear Your Recovery Proudly

Whether it is through ink or the clothes you wear, sober folks like to express their appreciation for their recovery. Some folks may look at it as being kind of preachy and pushy, but the bottom line is that you are loud and proud in your recovery. Besides, wearing a sandwich board would be hot and uncomfortable.

Ommmm...

As a recovering person, you are more than likely finding some time during the daily grind to find a quiet spot, sit comfortably, closing your eyes and just focusing on your breath. Mindful meditation is a relapse prevention staple, and the techniques are easy to master. Meditation does fancy robes or require insane flexibility. To meditate simply means finding a quiet spot and be one with your thoughts and reflect on the day.

You Make Plans

You know that you are a sober person when you can easily fill your daily schedule with recovery-based activities that are fun and help strengthen your recovery game. Whether it is meetings, hobbies or other activities, you don't have time to dwell on the pity pot and you surely don't have the energy to dwell on stinkin' thinkin'... for it is not in the planner for today–or any other day!

You Have Bank

In your active addiction, money was a tool that was used to feed an ego that ran amok–and as long as you felt good things such as paying bills and saving for the future could get a back seat or get thrown out the window entirely. A sign that you are a sober person is that you look at the money in your wallet and you find ways to make it work for you. The amount of cabbage that actually is in your wallet may be small, but it is yours and not going towards booze or dope so you have that going for you.

You Write It Down

When you are active in your recovery, you find creative and healthy outlet to channel your emotions—and journaling is one of those outlets. For those in recovery, the practice of journaling started in drug treatment, and it was a great tool to help you keep tabs on your day and was a great barometer in knowing what you were feeling at any given moment. If you continue to put pen to paper to help sort yourself out, it is yet another one of the signs that you are a sober person.

You Pay It Forward

One of the most important signs that you are a sober person is that you make paying it forward a huge part of your recovery program. Whether it is being a sponsor, being an ear to bend or a shoulder to cry on, or doing volunteer work, sobriety has shown you that sharing with others makes you feel good AND furthers your recovery.

Being Yourself

Ultimately, those who are sober embrace their true self, warts and all. You know that things aren't always pretty, but what you are is pretty awesome and that comes out for all to see.

The body cooperative notes:

- Most doctors only learn to fix sickness.
- Medical doctors have highjacked the healing space when in reality most have almost no knowledge about how to be healthy. Nutrition in not taught in medical schools.
- The average doctor gets about 2-hours of training in nutrition and virtually none in exercise or sleep. They learn little about the skills required to reflect on mental and physical health.
- "A good doctor's job is to provide health advice to people so that they can continue to enjoy that things they love without killing themselves any sooner than necessary." – Slattery
- We are individuals and are unique. There is no average human. Health is about the well-being of the whole person.
- The word doctor comes from the Latin word *Docere*, which means to teach.
- Patients are the most significant source of experience and knowledge for physicians.
- It's common for many generalist doctors to feel like they are just handing out medication. Which may help their performance numbers but its closer to putting a Band-Aid on the real problem.

- The problem doctors have is when they come across a health problem that they cannot quantify or that Big Pharma hasn't already created a medicine for an uncurable disease.
- Addiction can often fall into this category as its not a "real illness" in the sense that you cannot buy an over-the-counter cure or had your doctor write a prescription to cure all of the underlying problems that comes with addiction.
- When doctors cannot immediately solve your problem, this was something I dealt with personally, where I was just told to stop using, that I was simply stressed out and neurotic. Implying that someone is neurotic is the dumping ground of the diagnostic destitute and the wilderness for their patients, which is not helpful if you are the patient. I was sick and nobody knew what to do except make me feel guilty, which only made me feel worse. I couldn't even remember relapsing or using it most of the time. I understand that no one else was drugging me but it became very difficult to identify my triggers when I couldn't understand why I was using in the first place. I felt frightened and alone. My family gave me as much support as they could but it didn't seem to help. The only way I was able to avoid using was to travel to another country where NO2 is illegal. Compared to the

situation at home where there are 5 places that sell those 2-liter sized nitrous cans all within a few blocks of my house. Even the Dunkin donuts gas station sells them.

- The only recommendation that I was given by the doctors was to take large amounts of B-12. I was also suggested that I shouldn't drink or use any other intoxicates, however I still don't believe that the my nitrous abuse was related to anything else.
- I knew what was causing my illnesses but I couldn't stop using. I would remember dropping my kids off at school or being in a meeting at my office, then the next thing I would know it would be days later and I would wake up in my truck with gas cans everywhere. I was only able to track my usage by my credit card bill and counting the canisters in my vehicle when I would become conscious. I was averaging 10-15 thousand grams a day. This translates roughly into huffing 15 hours a day.
- In AA/NA they teach us that we are allergic to drugs and alcohol, the same way that people are allergic to peanuts or Gluten.
- Both my doctors and myself had been focusing on my symptoms and gut behaviors, entirely missing the fundamental question: why was I doing this to myself? I believe to this day that my entire body was out of balance, very

inflamed and extremely sick. This was solely my fault. I had a great childhood, wonderful parents, a great job, good friends, a luxury car, a beautiful wife and, most importantly, two amazing children.

- This is not a "poor me" account. It was a fact critical to who I am and perhaps what I do. I learned to survive, it made me tough, though the scars took a long time to heal.
- It became clear that this whole experience lead to an unbalanced neuro-immune system, and in turn an inflamed and distressed, foggy brain, along with a weakened body.
- I enhanced my psychological knowledge and skills, coming to understand why we continue to partake in habits that we know hurt us and why so many of us fail to stick with life choices that we all recognize will make us feel well. Its clear how our background, storyline, early/late traumas, injuries, and experiences can predict our own physical and mental health life story.
- So why trust me? I will tell you straight up because I have been to hell and back. A lifetime of addiction, bouncing between sickness and health. My hope in sharing my story and what I have learned will help you begin your journey to improved health and to save your life.

- This extends outside of addiction but applies to it directly, especially if you have been labeled as being an addict or having an illness without a known cause or explanation – this book is for you. You are not being neurotic or difficult, you have a very real medical condition!

Opioid use disorder (OUD) is defined as the chronic use of opioids that causes clinically significant distress or impairment. Symptoms of this disease include an overpowering desire to use opioids, increased opioid tolerance, and withdrawal syndrome when opioids are discontinued. Thus, OUD can range from dependence on opioids to addiction. OUD affects over 16 million people worldwide and over 2.1 million in the United States. Strikingly, there are as many patients using opioids regularly as there are patients diagnosed with obsessive-compulsive disorder, psoriatic arthritis, and epilepsy in the United States. More than 120,000 deaths worldwide every year are attributed to opioids. Examples of opioids include heroin (diacetylmorphine), morphine, codeine, fentanyl, and oxycodone.

A rise in the prevalence of OUD and opioid deaths lends to the importance of clinicians' appreciation for the complexity of OUD. OUD typically involves periods of exacerbation and remission, but the vulnerability to relapse occurs throughout a patient's lifetime. Stressful events, loss of economic stability, and relationship issues can increase the risk of relapse. Opioid addiction is similar to other chronic relapsing conditions; signs and symptoms can be severe, and treatment adherence is often problematic.

Mainstreaming Addiction Treatment (MAT) Act

The Mainstreaming Addiction Treatment (MAT) Act provision updates federal guidelines to expand the availability of evidence-based treatment to address the opioid epidemic. The MAT Act empowers all health care providers with a controlled substance certificate to prescribe buprenorphine for OUD, just as they prescribe other essential medications. The MAT Act is intended to help destigmatize a standard of care for OUD and strives to integrate substance use disorder treatment across healthcare settings.

As of December 2022, the MAT Act eliminated the DATA-Waiver (X-Waiver) program that was previously required to prescribe medications for the treatment of OUD. All DEA-registered practitioners with Schedule III prescribing authority may now prescribe buprenorphine for OUD in their practice if permitted by applicable state law. Prescribers previously registered with a DATA Waiver will receive a new DEA registration certificate reflecting this change without further action. Additionally, there are no longer limits on the number of patients with OUD that a practitioner may treat with buprenorphine or tracking of patients treated with buprenorphine required. Pharmacists can now dispense buprenorphine prescriptions using the prescribing authority's DEA number. Of note, prescribers are still required to comply with any applicable state limits regarding the treatment of patients with OUD. Information on State Opioid Treatment Authorities (SOTA) can be found at SAMHSA.gov.

Etiology

Opioid dependence and addiction are products of many biological, environmental, genetic, and psychosocial factors. Most opioids in use are prescribed, but many are also obtained illegally. After a relatively brief period, many patients taking opioids demonstrate opioid dependence. Opioid dependence can manifest as physical dependence, psychological dependence, or both. Opioid-dependent patients will experience withdrawal if opioids are stopped abruptly. Thus, many opioid-dependent patients will seek continued access to opioids, by legal or illegal means, to prevent withdrawal. Ongoing opioid dependence may lead to addiction and uncontrolled opioid use. OUD occurs in individuals from all educational and socioeconomic backgrounds. Patients at particular risk for OUD include those deficient in neurotransmitters such as dopamine or with first-degree relatives who have a substance abuse disorder. Patients who have been exposed to an environment that includes opioid use may also be more likely to develop OUD. Environmental risks for OUD include peer use of opioids or exposure to opioid analgesics due to a previous injury. Patients with a history of untreated depression, post-traumatic stress disorder, anxiety, or childhood trauma are also at risk for OUD.

Epidemiology

Over 16 million people worldwide and 3 million in the United States meet OUD criteria. Concerningly, OUD results in over 120,000 and 47,000 deaths per year worldwide and in the United States, respectively. In the United States, opioids have killed more people than any other drug in history. Recreational use of opioids was at its highest in 2010 and has gradually decreased as the opioid epidemic has gained attention in the United States. Up to 50% of patients on chronic opioid therapy meet the criteria for opioid use disorder.

The prevalence of opioid use and dependency varies by age and gender. Men are more likely to use and become dependent on opioids. Thus, men account for the majority of opioid-related overdoses. Women are prescribed opioids for analgesia more often than men. Opioid-related deaths are highest among individuals between the ages of 40 and 50 years, while heroin overdoses are most common among individuals between the ages of 20 and 30 years.

Pathophysiology

OUD develops along a continuum of opioid use. Physical dependence on opioids may develop rapidly and is likely the result of many changes in mu-opioid receptors, including receptor desensitization, internalization, and signaling abnormalities. Physical dependence is also responsible for withdrawal symptoms when opioids are stopped abruptly. Thus, physical dependence on opioids creates both positive and negative reinforcement for continued opioid use. Patients meet OUD criteria if their continued opioid use creates clinically significant impairment or distress. Clinically significant impairment and distress can manifest in several ways but are often the result of impairments in controlling opioid use and intense opioid cravings.

History and Physical

To make the diagnosis of OUD, the patient must meet the diagnostic criteria per the Diagnostic and Statistical Manual of Mental Disorders, Fifth Edition (DSM-5). Per the DSM-5, OUD is defined as repeated opioid use within 12 months leading to problems or distress with 2 or more of the following occurring:

1. Continued opioid use despite worsening physical or psychological health
2. Continued opioid use despite social and interpersonal consequences
3. Decreased social or recreational activities

4. Difficulty fulfilling professional duties at school or work
5. Excessive time is taken to obtain or recover from taking opioids
6. More opioids are taken than intended
7. Opioid cravings occur
8. Inability to decrease the amount of opioids used
9. Tolerance to opioids develops
10. Opioid use continues despite the dangers it poses to the user
11. Withdrawal occurs, or the user continues to take opioids to avoid withdrawal

The presence of 6 or more of these diagnostic criteria indicates severe OUD. The signs and symptoms of opioid use disorder include drug-seeking behavior, the presence of legal or social ramifications due to opioid use, multiple opioid prescriptions from different prescribers, opioid cravings, increased opioid usage over time, and symptoms of opioid withdrawal when stopping opioid use. Physical findings and complaints consistent with opioid withdrawal include muscle aches, diarrhea, rhinorrhea, nerve excitability, and chills with cessation of use.

Evaluation

A full social and mental health history should be a part of an initial evaluation for OUD. History of injuries, trauma, previous surgeries, and hospitalization may be crucial to the evaluation to identify gateways for opioid use. If the patient uses intravenous drugs, tests should be ordered to screen for HIV and hepatitis B and C. Urine drug screening for opioids should be performed before starting treatment for OUD and regularly with subsequent visits to evaluate the patient's compliance with treatment and abstinence from illicit opioid use.

Treatment / Management

The treatment of OUD improves physical and psychological conditions, reduces risks of overdose, and helps with the avoidance of criminal behavior and subsequent penalties. There are a variety of approaches to the rehabilitation and maintenance of patients with OUD. Rehabilitation begins with a cognitive behavioral approach similar to that used in the treatment of other chronic conditions. Maintenance programs include psychological support. Patients are encouraged and motivated to change through education, reward cooperation, and medications. The goal of cognitive behavioral therapy is to minimize drug relapses. Patients with OUD are encouraged to participate in self-help programs such as Narcotics Anonymous. The combination of education, motivational enhancement, and self-help assists patients to change how they think about the ways that opioids affect their lives. Group therapy helps maintain self-control and restraint for patients with OUD. Group therapy is also cost-effective compared to individualized therapy in treating OUD. Various forms of rehabilitation help patients recognize that change is possible. There is a need to decrease behaviors that perpetuate illicit drug use while developing new behaviors that diminish drug-related problems. Nonopioid drugs and physical therapy can provide a long-term solution to pain management instead of relying on the use of opioids, for example. Additionally, education about dealing with pain syndromes and minimizing opioid use can help build rapport and create realistic treatment goals. Cognitive behavioral therapy is most effective if combined with medications; however, there are mixed results on its effectiveness.

Opioid replacement, maintenance, or substitution therapy involves replacing the problematic opioid with a safer one. These alternative agents are prescribed under medical supervision. Medication-assisted treatment (MAT) and outpatient buprenorphine office therapy (OBOT) help the patient experience reduced symptoms of drug withdrawal and cravings and little or no euphoria. Opioid maintenance drugs help the patient experience reduced symptoms. Almost half of the patients can maintain abstinence from additional opioids while receiving replacement therapy.

The selection of which agent or agents to use for treatment can be simple or very complex, depending on patient-specific factors. Methadone, an oral mu-receptor agonist, is commonly used in opioid replacement. It has been widely used worldwide. In the US, outpatient methadone is offered only for specially monitored clinics. Patients with OUD with physiologic features of opioid withdrawal or who are likely to relapse are eligible to receive methadone from a clinic. The advantages of methadone treatment include reduced euphoric effects, decreased narcotic cravings, and reduced transmission of infectious diseases through avoidance of intravenous drug use. Methadone maintenance is non-sedating and is medically safe, provided there is no concomitant use of other prescription or illicit drugs. The maintenance phase can be attained with careful ramping of the dose upward. Consideration must be given to the long half-life of methadone, even if all of the symptoms of withdrawal, as well as the cravings, are not quickly abated. Other ancillary medications can be used to treat the symptoms as the dose of methadone is slowly increased. The length of the maintenance phase can last years to an entire lifetime. Tapering off methadone can take weeks or months, depending on the patient's level of opioid dependence.

An alternative oral, long-acting opioid for maintenance therapy is buprenorphine. Buprenorphine is a partial mu-receptor agonist. Similar to methadone, Buprenorphine is gradually ramped upwards to achieve an effective dose, and not all the symptoms of withdrawal can be immediately abated. It is crucial to ensure that the patient is in opioid withdrawal before the initiation of buprenorphine to avoid the occurrence of precipitated withdrawal. Buprenorphine is available as a sublingual tablet, sublingual film, buccal film, subcutaneous solution, transdermal patch, and intradermal implant. Sublingual tablets and films may also be combined with naloxone, a mu-opioid receptor antagonist. Naloxone is not absorbed orally and only exerts its action when injected into the bloodstream. Thus, the addition of naloxone to the buprenorphine formulation helps to deter abuse. Following induction and stabilization with sublingual tablets or the buccal film, subcutaneous solutions and intradermal implants may be used for lasting maintenance therapy.

There is no consensus among experts on whether methadone or buprenorphine therapy is superior in a broad population of patients with OUD.

Thus, the agent use should be based on patient-specific factors. The use of methadone maintenance may increase patient retention over buprenorphine. Additionally, methadone may treat withdrawal symptoms and cravings better than buprenorphine for patients who use fentanyl.

The length of treatment for OUD should also be individualized for each patient. Some clinicians attempt to discontinue medications for OUD after 1 year of treatment. Other clinicians suggest that treatment should be lifelong due to the risk of relapse and overdose death after patients stop treatment. If treatment is stopped, medications should be decreased slowly and adjusted if withdrawal symptoms are observed.

Naltrexone may also be used in patients with OUD. Naltrexone works by blocking opioid effects and helps maintain abstinence from opioids by antagonizing the mu-opioid receptor. Naltrexone may only be initiated when the patient is free of physiological opioid dependence, and at least seven days without acute withdrawal symptoms are required before starting the medication. Both oral and intramuscular naltrexone are superior to placebo in maintaining abstinence from opioids, but the intramuscular form may be more effective. The intramuscular form may also offer better compliance due to monthly administrations. Intramuscular naltrexone is FDA-approved for opioid dependence, and naltrexone administration following completion of treatment with buprenorphine has shown to be an effective treatment in OUD.

Many other medications are used adjunctively to treat OUD. Clonidine may abate withdrawal symptoms while the dose of methadone or buprenorphine is being adjusted. Tizanidine helps decrease anxiety as well as muscle pain associated with opioid withdrawal. Bupropion is used to combat the symptoms of anxiety. Diarrhea, nausea, and vomiting are treated with loperamide and ondansetron, respectively.

Differential Diagnosis

The differential diagnosis of OUD includes malingering and other substance abuse disorders. Chronic pain disorders and untreated mental health issues may also appear similar to OUD. Evaluation and identification of the underlying medical and mental health disorders are of the utmost importance in making a definitive diagnosis of OUD. Often, OUD is diagnosed in addition to other substance abuse and mental health disorders.

Prognosis

The diagnosis of OUD helps clinicians to mitigate risks for patients taking chronic opioids. Clinicians should offer naloxone to all patients with OUD.

Patients are at the highest risk for opioid-related death in the first 4 weeks of OUD treatment and for 4 weeks after treatment ends. Thus, close contact with the patient should be maintained both during and after treatment.

OUD treatment reduces the incidence of long-term opioid addiction while decreasing illegal opioid use and mortality. Crimes associated with drugs and the expense of dealing with HIV, sepsis, and other medical complications are also decreased. Specifically, methadone treatment is associated with a 50% reduction in all-cause mortality, as well as a 50% reduction in the incidence of hepatitis C. Methadone therapy has also been shown to decrease drug-related crimes and illicit drug use, improve social interactions, and increase rates of retention in rehabilitation programs.

Complications

Addiction is the most severe complication of OUD. Addiction to opioids is the continued use of these drugs despite adverse consequences or events. Opioid addiction occurs by sensitizing the drug-reward system and amplifying compulsive drug-seeking. Specifically, chronic opioid use affects the orbitofrontal area, which is essential for regulating anxiety, emotional responses, and reward-related behaviors. Additionally, opioid addiction affects every aspect of a person's life. Legal trouble, loss of personal relationships, and significant morbidity and mortality are all consequences of opioid addiction. Opioid withdrawal is also a significant complication of OUD. Opioid withdrawal onset varies with the type of opioid used. Heroin withdrawal begins in as little as five hours, whereas methadone withdrawal may occur 2 to 3 days following the last ingestion. The duration of opioid withdrawal symptoms varies greatly by patient. Thus, symptoms may last for a few days or persist for weeks. Finally, opioid overdose may occur as a result of OUD. The risk of overdose in untreated patients with OUD is high, but there is still a significant risk of overdose in patients who have received treatment. The time of highest risk for treated patients is the period between detoxification and the start of maintenance therapy. The use and acceptance of cognitive behavioral therapy may decrease this risk. Sadly, however, the mortality rate for patients on chronic opioids remains extremely high.

Deterrence and Patient Education

Methadone and buprenorphine should be considered for patients with OUD to minimize the risk of death. Naloxone is used in the acute treatment of an opiate overdose and can be given subcutaneously, intramuscularly, intravenously, intranasally, or by inhalation. It is reasonable to prescribe naloxone to any patient with OUD. Naloxone prescriptions should also be considered for a more general population of patients taking chronic opioids. Finally, the involvement of an addiction or pain medicine specialist in the care of patients with OUD is essential to the development of a comprehensive and effective treatment plan.

Enhancing Healthcare Team Outcomes

Appropriate treatment of OUD requires an interprofessional approach. Specifically, cognitive and behavioral therapies need to be supported by medical intervention to reduce the chance of withdrawal, relapse, and overdose. An interprofessional team, including physicians or advanced practice providers, nurses, pharmacists, therapists, and other addiction and substance use professionals, is responsible for coordinating OUD care. The tenets of comprehensive OUD care include:

1. Timely diagnosis of OUD

2. Discussion of the OUD diagnosis (focusing on the immediate and long-term effects of opioids on morbidity and mortality)

3. Treatment of the underlying conditions associated with OUD (ie, cognitive behavioral therapy and antidepressants for major depressive disorder)

4. Prescription of naloxone for the treatment of overdose

5. Prescription of opioid replacement therapy or referral to an addiction medicine specialist to manage opioid replacement therapy
6. Referral to a rehabilitation program to promote cognitive and behavioral changes

Physicians, advanced practice providers, and pharmacists all play a role in recognizing and diagnosing OUD. While physicians and advanced practice providers may make the formal diagnosis of OUD, nurses and pharmacists may be the first to notice opioid misuse. Nurses may detect opioid misuse through patient screening and interviews. Pharmacists may identify patterns of opioid misuse by noting the duration of use, the receipt of opioid prescriptions from multiple providers, and the number of early refill requests. All team members play a vital role in the treatment of OUD. Physicians and advanced practice providers prescribe medications for OUD, including buprenorphine under the MAT Act, and make referrals for cognitive behavioral therapies. Nurses assist with coordinating OUD therapies and educating patients on the importance of therapy adherence. Pharmacists and addiction medicine specialists provide recommendations to optimize OUD medication therapies and promote adherence to cognitive behavioral therapies.

Therapists and other addiction and substance abuse professionals carry out cognitive behavioral therapies and promote adherence to medical therapies. Ultimately, a successful, interprofessional approach will optimize OUD therapy for patients. Effective communication and coordination among all healthcare team members are integral to a successful approach. Additionally, the healthcare team should empower family members and members of the lay public to support the tenets of OUD care. This may further improve a patient's chances of successful OUD management.

References

1.

Vallersnes OM, Jacobsen D, Ekeberg Ø, Brekke M. Mortality, morbidity and follow-up after acute poisoning by substances of abuse: A prospective observational cohort study. Scand J Public Health. 2019 Jun;47(4):452-461. [PubMed]

2.

Chang HY, Kharrazi H, Bodycombe D, Weiner JP, Alexander GC. Healthcare costs and utilization associated with high-risk prescription opioid use: a retrospective cohort study. BMC Med. 2018 May 16;16(1):69. [PMC free article] [PubMed]

3.

Brat GA, Agniel D, Beam A, Yorkgitis B, Bicket M, Homer M, Fox KP, Knecht DB, McMahill-Walraven CN, Palmer N, Kohane I. Postsurgical prescriptions for opioid naive patients and association with overdose and misuse: retrospective cohort study. BMJ. 2018 Jan 17;360:j5790. [PMC free article] [PubMed]

4.

Dick DM, Agrawal A. The genetics of alcohol and other drug dependence. Alcohol Res Health. 2008;31(2):111-8. [PMC free article] [PubMed]

5.

Sharma B, Bruner A, Barnett G, Fishman M. Opioid Use Disorders. Child Adolesc Psychiatr Clin N Am. 2016 Jul;25(3):473-87. [PMC free article] [PubMed]

6.

Theisen K, Jacobs B, Macleod L, Davies B. The United States opioid epidemic: a review of the surgeon's contribution to it and health policy initiatives. BJU Int. 2018 Nov;122(5):754-759. [PubMed]

7.

Højsted J, Sjøgren P. Addiction to opioids in chronic pain patients: a literature review. Eur J Pain. 2007 Jul;11(5):490-518. [PubMed]

8.

Christie MJ. Cellular neuroadaptations to chronic opioids: tolerance, withdrawal and addiction. Br J Pharmacol. 2008 May;154(2):384-96. [PMC free article] [PubMed]

9.

Rich MM, Wenner P. Sensing and expressing homeostatic synaptic plasticity. Trends Neurosci. 2007 Mar;30(3):119-25. [PubMed]

10.

Volkow ND, Blanco C. The changing opioid crisis: development, challenges and opportunities. Mol Psychiatry. 2021 Jan;26(1):218-233. [PMC free article] [PubMed]

11.

John WS, Zhu H, Mannelli P, Schwartz RP, Subramaniam GA, Wu LT. Prevalence, patterns, and correlates of multiple substance use disorders among adult primary care patients. Drug Alcohol Depend. 2018 Jun 01;187:79-87. [PMC free article] [PubMed]

12.

Ober AJ, Watkins KE, McCullough CM, Setodji CM, Osilla K, Hunter SB. Patient predictors of substance use disorder treatment initiation in primary care. J Subst Abuse Treat. 2018 Jul;90:64-72. [PMC free article] [PubMed]

13.

LeFevre ML., U.S. Preventive Services Task Force. Screening for hepatitis B virus infection in nonpregnant adolescents and adults: U.S. Preventive Services Task Force recommendation statement. Ann Intern Med. 2014 Jul 01;161(1):58-66. [PubMed]

14.

Moyer VA., U.S. Preventive Services Task Force. Screening for hepatitis C virus infection in adults: U.S. Preventive Services Task Force recommendation statement. Ann Intern Med. 2013 Sep 03;159(5):349-57. [PubMed]

15.

Moyer VA., U.S. Preventive Services Task Force*. Screening for HIV: U.S. Preventive Services Task Force Recommendation Statement. Ann Intern Med. 2013 Jul 02;159(1):51-60. [PubMed]

16.

Johnson RE, Strain EC, Amass L. Buprenorphine: how to use it right. Drug Alcohol Depend. 2003 May 21;70(2 Suppl):S59-77. [PubMed]

17.

Moberg K. The role of managed care professionals and pharmacists in combating opioid abuse. Am J Manag Care. 2018 May;24(10 Suppl):S215-S223. [PubMed]

18.

Szalavitz M, Rigg KK. The Curious (Dis)Connection between the Opioid Epidemic and Crime. Subst Use Misuse. 2017 Dec 06;52(14):1927-1931. [PubMed]

19.

Fals-Stewart W, O'Farrell TJ. Behavioral family counseling and naltrexone for male opioid-dependent patients. J Consult Clin Psychol. 2003 Jun;71(3):432-42. [PubMed]

20.

Gossop M, Stewart D, Marsden J. Attendance at Narcotics Anonymous and Alcoholics Anonymous meetings, frequency of attendance and substance use outcomes after residential treatment for drug dependence: a 5-year follow-up study. Addiction. 2008 Jan;103(1):119-25. [PubMed]

21.

Galanter M. Combining medically assisted treatment and Twelve-Step programming: a perspective and review. Am J Drug Alcohol Abuse. 2018;44(2):151-159. [PubMed]

22.

Fals-Stewart W, O'Farrell TJ, Birchler GR. Behavioral couples therapy for substance abuse: rationale, methods, and findings. Sci Pract Perspect. 2004 Aug;2(2):30-41. [PMC free article] [PubMed]

23.

Meyers RJ, Miller WR, Hill DE, Tonigan JS. Community reinforcement and family training (CRAFT): engaging unmotivated drug users in treatment. J Subst Abuse. 1998;10(3):291-308. [PubMed]

24.

Fiellin DA, Barry DT, Sullivan LE, Cutter CJ, Moore BA, O'Connor PG, Schottenfeld RS. A randomized trial of cognitive behavioral therapy in primary care-based buprenorphine. Am J Med. 2013 Jan;126(1):74.e11-7. [PMC free article] [PubMed]

25.

Strain EC, Stitzer ML, Liebson IA, Bigelow GE. Dose-response effects of methadone in the treatment of opioid dependence. Ann Intern Med. 1993 Jul 01;119(1):23-7. [PubMed]

26.

Gibson A, Degenhardt L, Mattick RP, Ali R, White J, O'Brien S. Exposure to opioid maintenance treatment reduces long-term mortality. Addiction. 2008 Mar;103(3):462-8. [PubMed]

27.

Faggiano F, Vigna-Taglianti F, Versino E, Lemma P. Methadone maintenance at different dosages for opioid dependence. Cochrane Database Syst Rev. 2003;(3):CD002208. [PubMed]

28.

Johnson RE, Chutuape MA, Strain EC, Walsh SL, Stitzer ML, Bigelow GE. A comparison of levomethadyl acetate, buprenorphine, and methadone for opioid dependence. N Engl J Med. 2000 Nov 02;343(18):1290-7. [PubMed]

29.

Kakko J, Svanborg KD, Kreek MJ, Heilig M. 1-year retention and social function after buprenorphine-assisted relapse prevention treatment for heroin dependence in Sweden: a randomised, placebo-controlled trial. Lancet. 2003 Feb 22;361(9358):662-8. [PubMed]

30.

Mattick RP, Breen C, Kimber J, Davoli M. Buprenorphine maintenance versus placebo or methadone maintenance for opioid dependence. Cochrane Database Syst Rev. 2014 Feb 06;2014(2):CD002207. [PMC free article] [PubMed]

31.

Ma J, Bao YP, Wang RJ, Su MF, Liu MX, Li JQ, Degenhardt L, Farrell M, Blow FC, Ilgen M, Shi J, Lu L. Effects of medication-assisted treatment on mortality among opioids users: a systematic review and meta-analysis. Mol Psychiatry. 2019 Dec;24(12):1868-1883. [PubMed]

32.

Kakko J, Heilig M, Sarman I. Buprenorphine and methadone treatment of opiate dependence during pregnancy: comparison of fetal growth and neonatal outcomes in two consecutive case series. Drug Alcohol Depend. 2008 Jul 01;96(1-2):69-78. [PubMed]

33.

Senay EC, Dorus W, Goldberg F, Thornton W. Withdrawal from methadone maintenance. Rate of withdrawal and expectation. Arch Gen Psychiatry. 1977 Mar;34(3):361-7. [PubMed]

34.

Minozzi S, Amato L, Vecchi S, Davoli M, Kirchmayer U, Verster A. Oral naltrexone maintenance treatment for opioid dependence. Cochrane Database Syst Rev. 2011 Apr 13;2011(4):CD001333. [PMC free article] [PubMed]

35.

Edelman EJ, Oldfield BJ, Tetrault JM. Office-Based Addiction Treatment in Primary Care: Approaches That Work. Med Clin North Am. 2018 Jul;102(4):635-652. [PubMed]

36.

Fudala PJ, Bridge TP, Herbert S, Williford WO, Chiang CN, Jones K, Collins J, Raisch D, Casadonte P, Goldsmith RJ, Ling W, Malkerneker U, McNicholas L, Renner J, Stine S, Tusel D., Buprenorphine/Naloxone Collaborative Study Group. Office-based treatment of opiate addiction with a sublingual-tablet formulation of buprenorphine and naloxone. N Engl J Med. 2003 Sep 04;349(10):949-58. [PubMed]

37.

Dowell D, Haegerich TM, Chou R. CDC Guideline for Prescribing Opioids for Chronic Pain--United States, 2016. JAMA. 2016 Apr 19;315(15):1624-45. [PMC free article] [PubMed]

38.

Coffin PO, Behar E, Rowe C, Santos GM, Coffa D, Bald M, Vittinghoff E. Nonrandomized Intervention Study of Naloxone Coprescription for Primary Care Patients Receiving Long-Term Opioid Therapy for Pain. Ann Intern Med. 2016 Aug 16;165(4):245-52. [PMC free article] [PubMed]

39.

National Academies of Sciences, Engineering, and Medicine; Health and Medicine Division; Board on Health Sciences Policy; Committee on Pain Management and Regulatory Strategies to Address Prescription Opioid Abuse. Pain Management and the Opioid Epidemic: Balancing Societal and Individual Benefits and Risks of Prescription Opioid Use. Phillips JK, Ford MA, Bonnie RJ, editors. National Academies Press (US); Washington (DC): Jul 13, 2017. [PubMed]

40.

Gandhi DH, Jaffe JH, McNary S, Kavanagh GJ, Hayes M, Currens M. Short-term outcomes after brief ambulatory opioid detoxification with buprenorphine in young heroin users. Addiction. 2003 Apr;98(4):453-62. [PubMed]

41.

Sordo L, Barrio G, Bravo MJ, Indave BI, Degenhardt L, Wiessing L, Ferri M, Pastor-Barriuso R. Mortality risk during and after opioid substitution treatment: systematic review and meta-analysis of cohort studies. BMJ. 2017 Apr 26;357:j1550. [PMC free article] [PubMed]

42.

Fullerton CA, Kim M, Thomas CP, Lyman DR, Montejano LB, Dougherty RH, Daniels AS, Ghose SS, Delphin-Rittmon ME. Medication-assisted treatment with methadone: assessing the evidence. Psychiatr Serv. 2014 Feb 01;65(2):146-57. [PubMed]

43.

Sorensen JL, Copeland AL. Drug abuse treatment as an HIV prevention strategy: a review. Drug Alcohol Depend. 2000 Apr 01;59(1):17-31. [PubMed]

44.

Clinical Guidelines for Withdrawal Management and Treatment of Drug Dependence in Closed Settings. World Health Organization; Geneva: 2009. [PubMed]

45.

Hser YI, Mooney LJ, Saxon AJ, Miotto K, Bell DS, Zhu Y, Liang D, Huang D. High Mortality Among Patients With Opioid Use Disorder in a Large Healthcare System. J Addict Med. 2017 Jul/Aug;11(4):315-319. [PMC free article] [PubMed]

46.

Zhang X, Marchand C, Sullivan B, Klass EM, Wagner KD. Naloxone access for Emergency Medical Technicians: An evaluation of a training program in rural communities. Addict Behav. 2018 Nov;86:79-85. [PubMed]

47.

Kinsman JM, Robinson K. National Systematic Legal Review of State Policies on Emergency Medical Services Licensure Levels' Authority to Administer Opioid Antagonists. Prehosp Emerg Care. 2018 Sep-Oct;22(5):650-654. [PubMed]

48.

Matthew O. Howard, Frank A. Daniels Professor for Human Services Policy Information at the University of North Carolina at Chapel Hill, also collaborated on this project.

49.

Tsipursky, G. (2019). Never Go With Your Gut: How Pioneering Leaders Make the Best Decisions and Avoid Business Disasters. Newburyport, MA: Career Press.

www.ingramcontent.com/pod-product-compliance
Lightning Source LLC
Chambersburg PA
CBHW070345230526
45471CB00006B/2433